Clinical Textbook for
Nurses

Barbara McDonald

Veterinary

veterinary medicine is a medical specialty that focuses on the prevention, control, diagnosis, and treatment of diseases that affect the health of domestic and wild animals as well as the prevention of the transmission of animal diseases to humans. Veterinary medicine is also known as veterinary science. By keeping an eye on and taking care of the health of animals that produce food, veterinarians ensure that people have a safe supply of food

Animal doctors have been around since the beginning of recorded history, and veterinary medicine was already a speciality in Babylonia and Egypt in 2000 BCE. The ancient Greeks had a group of doctors they called "horse-doctors." In modern times, the field is now known by the Latin term "veterinarius," which means "pertaining to beast of burden." Veterinarians today work in a variety of settings, including private and corporate clinical practice, academic programs, private industry, public health, the military, and the government. Other veterinary medicine professionals, such as veterinary technicians and veterinary nurses, frequently assist them in their work.

Numerous significant advancements in animal and human health can be attributed to veterinary medicine. Reduced animal sources of human exposure to brucellosis and tuberculosis are also included. Numerous diseases affecting companion animals (also known as pets) can now be prevented with safe and effective vaccines, such as canine and feline panleukopenia, respectively. The first vaccine against cancer was made for chickens to control Marek's disease. Surgical procedures like hip-joint replacement and organ transplants were developed by veterinarians and later successfully applied to humans.

The wide range of animal species presents a significant obstacle for veterinary medicine. The health requirements of domestic animals, such as cats, dogs, chickens, horses, cows, sheep, pigs, and goats, are addressed by veterinarians. wildlife; animals in zoos; avian pets; also, decorative fish. Animals are treated in a variety of sizes, from newborn hamsters to adult elephants. Their economic values also vary, from the unquantifiable value of pet animal companionship to the high monetary value of a successful racehorse. This variety of domesticated and wild animals needs special skills and knowledge to be used as medicines.

There are approximately 450 veterinary degree programs around the world that are approved by the government of a country or the World Health Organization (WHO). Only about one third of these programs award a doctoral degree, and the level of veterinary training varies greatly from country to country. A veterinarian's professional education typically consists of two phases. Anatomy, physiology, pathology, pharmacology, toxicology, nutrition, microbiology, and public health are just some of the preclinical sciences covered in the first, or basic science, phase, which entails classroom instruction and laboratory work. Infectious and noninfectious diseases, diagnostic and clinical pathology, obstetrics, radiology, anesthesiology, surgery, and practice management are all covered in the second phase, which focuses on the clinical sciences. Students also get hands-on clinical experience in the college's veterinary teaching hospital. Students can interact with animal owners, treat sick animals, and carry out surgery during the clinical experience. Graduate veterinarians on the faculty are in charge of supervising student activities in the clinical setting. Graduate veterinarians have access to a number of significant opportunities for additional education. Veterinarians are able to acquire clinical proficiency in one or two medical specialties through internship (one-year) and residency (two to five years) programs. Advanced degree programs are another option for veterinarians who have graduated. Although some people seek advanced degrees in fields like business, the majority of advanced study is focused on medicine.

The majority of clinical-practice veterinarians only treat companion animals in the animal hospital or clinic of their practice. A small percentage only treat horses or animals that produce food, frequently traveling to the animal's location in a vehicle designed for field veterinary care. The majority of the remaining clinical practitioners work in mixed practices, which handle both domesticated small animals and large ones like cattle or horses. Services for special species like ornamental fish, caged birds, and reptiles are provided by some small-animal practices. Work may be restricted to surgery, dentistry, dermatology, or ophthalmology by some practices. There has been an increase in the number of corporately owned animal hospitals, many of which also offer pet supplies for sale.

Academic veterinarians oversee veterinary colleges' basic and clinical science programs. In addition, they carry out research at the fundamental and clinical levels, the latter of which may involve putting brand-new instrumentation technologies to use in the process of diagnosing and treating animal diseases. Endoscopy, nuclear scintigraphy, ultrasonography, computed tomography (CT) scans, and magnetic resonance imaging (MRI) are all included. referred to as nuclear magnetic resonance).

In areas like animal health monitoring in large commercial animal production programs, biomedical research, and product marketing, veterinary medicine and private industry interact. Toxicology, laboratory animal medicine, pathology, molecular biology, and genetic engineering are among the fields in which industry vets specialize. In the development, safety testing, and clinical evaluation of drugs, chemicals, and biological products like vaccines and antibiotics for humans and animals, pharmaceutical companies employ veterinarians.

Animal welfare, environmental protection, agricultural research, food and drug safety, public health, and food-animal inspection are all areas in which veterinarians are employed by both federal and state governments. Public-health veterinarians, for instance, assess the food-processing facilities, restaurants, and water supplies' safety. Additionally, they assist in the management of human and animal disease outbreaks. Due to the growing threat posed by bioterrorism, veterinarians now play a crucial role in preventing the use of zoonotic organisms as weapons and safeguarding the food supply for humans and animals. Aerospace also employs veterinarians; For instance, they have served as members of US space shuttle crews and served as scientific advisors on the use of animals in the space program. Biomedical research, caring for military dogs, and food inspection and communicable disease monitoring and control programs are all performed by veterinarians in the military.

What is the job of a veterinarian?

What exactly is a vet?

A veterinarian is a medical professional who focuses on providing animal patients with medical care. They are responsible for diagnosing and treating injuries, diseases, and illnesses in a variety of animals, including livestock, wildlife, and household pets. In addition, veterinarians carry out routine procedures, vaccinations, and examinations in order to safeguard the well-being and health of animals.

Veterinarians educate pet owners and those who take care of animals about the best ways to feed and care for their animals. They might also work in research to come up with new technologies and treatments that will help animals live better lives. By monitoring and controlling the spread of diseases that can be transmitted between animals and humans, veterinarians play a crucial role in public health.

The health and well-being of animals, which has a significant impact on human health, is crucially maintained by veterinarians. Veterinarians contribute to the well-being and success of animals by providing preventative care, diagnosing and treating diseases, and addressing health issues. This is essential not only for the animals themselves but also for the people who interact with them, whether they serve as companions, farm animals, or food sources.

Duties and Responsibilities

For people who are passionate about animal health and welfare, becoming a veterinarian can be a rewarding and fulfilling career choice. Some of their responsibilities include the following:

Identifying and treating animal ailments, injuries, and diseases: Veterinarians diagnose and treat a wide range of animal medical conditions through physical examinations, medical histories, and diagnostic tests like X-rays and blood work.

Executing surgical operations: From routine spaying and neutering to more involved surgeries to treat injuries or illnesses, veterinarians perform surgical procedures.

Preventative care and medication administration: In order to maintain an animal's health and well-being, veterinarians prescribe medications and provide preventive services like vaccination, parasite control, and dental care.

Providing pet owners and caregivers with information: Veterinarians teach pet people and creature overseers on legitimate creature care practices, sustenance, and dependable pet possession.

Investing in research: In order to improve animal health and well-being, some veterinarians participate in research to develop novel technologies and treatments.

Keeping an eye on and stopping the spread of diseases: By monitoring and controlling the spread of diseases that can be transmitted between animals and humans, veterinarians play a crucial role in public health.

Providing care in an emergency: Animals that have been injured or are in critical condition require immediate medical attention from veterinarians.

Animal welfare advice: Concerns for the well-being of animals, such as cruelty, neglect, and animal abuse, are addressed by veterinarians.

Different kinds of veterinarians

Veterinary medicine is a broad field that includes many different specialties. While all veterinarians receive a comprehensive education in animal health and welfare, some opt to pursue specialized training and education. These specialists in veterinary medicine provide specialized care to animals in need in a variety of settings, including private practices and research facilities.

Veterinarians of Small Animals: These veterinarians treat domesticated animals like cats, dogs, and other small animals.

Huge Creature Veterinarians: These veterinarians are experts in taking care of farm animals like horses, cows, sheep, and pigs.

Veterinarians for exotic animals: The care of exotic animals, such as birds, reptiles, and other non-traditional pets, is the area of expertise of these veterinarians.

Veterinarians for Wildlife: These veterinarians take care of animals that live in the wild, such as those in zoos, wildlife reserves, and natural habitats.

Veterinarians for horses: These veterinarians treat horses and other equine species exclusively.

Veterinarians in critical and emergency care: These veterinarians specialize in providing urgent care to animals in need and work in emergency clinics.

Surgeons for Animals: These veterinarians are experts in animal surgery, from simple procedures like spaying and neutering to more complicated operations.

Behaviorists for pets: Animal behavioral problems are the area of expertise of these veterinarians.

Veterinarians in Public Health: These veterinarians specialize in human and animal disease control and prevention in public health settings.

Pathologists for animals: These veterinarians frequently participate in research and diagnosis due to their specialization in the study of animal diseases.

What is a veterinarian's workplace like?

A veterinarian's work environment can be very different from one practice to the next. Private clinics, animal hospitals, research facilities, zoos, and even farms are all places veterinarians can work.

The veterinarian typically works in an exam room or treatment area in a private clinic or animal hospital, where they perform physical examinations, diagnose illnesses, and perform surgical procedures. They might also have an office where they can look over patient records, talk to patients, and run the clinic's business.

Veterinarians frequently work in laboratories at research facilities, where they carry out experiments and research to improve animal health and medicine. They might collaborate with other scientists to develop novel technologies and treatments and work with a variety of animal species.

In zoological parks or aquariums, zoo veterinarians are in charge of the health and welfare of the animals under their care. They may conduct routine examinations, provide preventative care, diagnose and treat diseases, and, if necessary, carry out surgeries or other procedures.

Farm animal veterinarians frequently travel to various locations to provide medical care and advise farmers on animal health and production issues. They might work with cows, pigs, and chickens, and they might be in charge of keeping an eye on the health of the herd and treating individual animals as needed.

What misconceptions do you hear about working as a veterinarian?

It is essential to dispel a number of misconceptions regarding the profession of veterinarian. Among the most prevalent misconceptions are:

Only dogs and cats are treated by vets: Although many veterinarians deal with dogs and cats, the practice of veterinary medicine encompasses a much broader range of animals. Animals that veterinarians can treat include wildlife, exotic animals, and livestock.

It's easy to become a veterinarian: The field of veterinary medicine is hard and requires a lot of education and training. An excellent understanding of anatomy, physiology, pharmacology, and other fields is essential for veterinarians. In addition, in order to work with both animals and their owners, they need to have excellent interpersonal and communication skills.

There are no two veterinarians alike: Because the field of veterinary medicine is comprised of numerous subdisciplines, not all veterinarians possess the same level of education or expertise. For instance, a veterinarian with a specialty in small animal medicine will have different abilities and knowledge than one with a specialty in equine medicine.

Private practices are where veterinarians only work: There are numerous other career options for veterinarians, despite the fact that many of them work in private practices. Veterinarians can work in government, academia, and research, among other fields.

What's good and bad about being a veterinarian? For people who are passionate about animal health and welfare, becoming a veterinarian is a rewarding career choice. The diagnosis and treatment of diseases, the provision of preventative care, and the enhancement of animals' lives all depend on veterinarians. However, as with any profession, pursuing a career in veterinary medicine has both advantages and disadvantages.

Pros

Possibility of working with animals: The opportunity to daily work with animals is one of the best aspects of being a veterinarian. If you're passionate about animal health and welfare, this can be a very rewarding experience.

Beneficial effects on pets and their owners: Animals' health and well-being are greatly enhanced by veterinarians. This may have a beneficial effect not only on the animals themselves but also on their owners, who may experience feelings of relief and appreciation for the care they have received.

Numerous career options: There are a lot of sub-disciplines in veterinary medicine, so there are many different career paths. Small, large, exotic, and even wild animals can all be treated by a veterinarian.

Demand for veterinarians is high: The job outlook for veterinarians is positive, with a projected 16% growth rate between 2019 and 2029, according to the Bureau of Labor Statistics. As a result of this high demand, salaries can be competitive and stable.

Cons

Impact on emotions: It can be emotionally taxing to work with sick or injured animals, and veterinarians may experience compassion fatigue or burnout.

Hourly work and erratic schedules: Veterinarians may be expected to work long hours, including on holidays and weekends. Additionally, situations that call for veterinarians to be on call or to work extended hours may occur.

a lot of student debt: The cost of veterinary schooling can be quite high, and many recent graduates might end up with a lot of debt from student loans. Their career choices and financial security may be affected by this.

difficile choices: Veterinarians may have to make difficult decisions about things like euthanasia or end-of-life care, which can be hard on the heart and can make them feel guilty or anxious.

In conclusion, if you have a passion for animal health and welfare, becoming a veterinarian can be a rewarding and fulfilling career choice. But before taking this route, it's important to weigh the benefits and drawbacks because it can be emotionally taxing and requires a lot of education and training.

How much time does it take to become a vet?

Typically, it takes several years of education and training to become a veterinarian. The individual circumstances, such as the availability of prerequisite courses, admission requirements, and program length, may influence the timeline. Here is an outline of the ordinary advances expected to turn into a veterinarian:

Earn your bachelor's degree: Typically, this requires full-time study for four years.

Follow through with essential courses: These classes can take anywhere from one to two more years to complete and typically include math, physics, biology, and chemistry.

Study veterinary medicine: This typically requires full-time study for four years.

Get a license: To become licensed to practice in the United States, individuals who have completed veterinary school must pass the North American Veterinary Licensing Exam (NAVLE).

A minimum of seven to eight years of education and training are required to become a veterinarian, but individual circumstances may alter the timeline. Additionally, the timeline may be extended by additional years if some veterinarians decide to pursue additional training or education in specialized fields.

Veterinarian The AV must be a graduate of an accredited veterinary medicine school or have an equivalent formal education, have experience in the care and management of animals, and have direct or delegated authority over activities involving animals at the facility.

Case Scenario: Shared Strategies to Improve Human and Animal Health Shared Behavioral Dangers A veterinarian is performing a routine checkup on a dog that is three years old. She observes that the dog is now significantly overweight and has gained 10 pounds in the past 18 months. In addition, the owner is corpulent. The veterinarian finds out when they inquire about the dog's exercise routines that the dog rarely walks and spends most of its time in a small yard. The vet asks the owner if he or she has thought about getting more exercise for himself. The owner confirms that he used to regularly jog, but there are currently no sidewalks in the suburban development where they live. The owner is informed of a nearby dog park with a perimeter walking path that is within a 10-minute drive, despite the veterinarian's agreement that this makes it more difficult to take the dog for walks. The dog's diet is modified, and the owner is advised to have his health care provider evaluate him before beginning an exercise program. She writes a letter to the healthcare provider with the owner's permission.

The patient's nurse practitioner calls the veterinarian the following week to express her appreciation for the veterinarian's assistance in motivating the patient to begin an exercise program. Both the patient and the dog's nurse practitioner and veterinarian agree to set exercise and weight loss goals and separate reinforcements for the healthy behavior change. In addition, they agree to collaborate on a letter to the town mayor highlighting the necessity of constructing a walking path in the patient's neighborhood to improve the health of both people and their companion animals. Although it takes some time, the walking paths are eventually built, in part thanks to the efforts of health professionals.

Law and Regulations in Israel Concerning the Use of Animals in Biological and Medical Research Veterinary Care the Guide2 standards (pages 106–124) govern Israel's veterinary treatment of laboratory animals.

The Guide outlines the roles of the AV in accordance with the Law. This increases the AV's authority and makes him the animal's final voice regarding its health and destiny. Animal welfare and health oversight are the responsibility of the AV; offer medical treatment;

ward off diseases; minimizing the suffering of animals prior to, during, and following the experiments; when necessary, put animals to sleep; and teach employees about these issues.

For the purposes of the law, the AV must be a diplomat in LAM or a veterinarian with authorization from the National Director of Veterinary Services and Animal Health—Ministry of Agriculture. The Gathering, in a joint effort with the Public Overseer of Veterinary Administrations and Creature Wellbeing — Service of Horticulture, set certification measures for veterinarians who are not negotiators in LAM and concluded that this approval will be restricted for a period not surpassing a long time from the primary endorsement. After this time, applications for renewal should be sent to the accreditation committee.

Infectious Disease Scenarios Case Study 2

A 7-year-old neutered female cat was brought in for toxoplasmosis serologic testing and (reluctant) possible euthanasia by a public health veterinarian who was also a relief clinical veterinarian. The owner of the cat was the spouse of a cancer patient. He or she was worried that the husband or wife was receiving immunosuppressive chemotherapy, which put them at high risk of contracting toxoplasmosis from their pet. The veterinarian explained the toxoplasmosis life cycle, the human and cat epidemic, and how a positive serology could actually be protective. Due to the fact that the cat was only kept indoors, was exclusively fed a commercial diet, and had never hunted in its life, the owner refused both euthanasia and serologic testing. The cat's risk of contracting the parasite was reduced because there was no evidence of rats or mice in the house. However, the spouse's love of gardening raises the risk of contracting toxoplasmosis significantly. Fortunately, the patient washed thoroughly afterward and always used gloves. The veterinarian and the feline proprietor examined extra toxoplasmosis openness decrease, including legitimate treatment of crude meats and washing crude food sources. The cat's owner and the veterinarian agreed that the owner would clean the litter box, have the cat examined for overall health every six months, and bring the cat in for treatment and prevention of zoonotic diseases in the event of diarrhea or signs of respiratory disease.

Controlled Substances Laboratory Animal Care

Veterinarians Due to their inherent responsibilities for managing animal care and health as well as regulatory compliance, laboratory animal veterinarians and animal care program directors have historically provided and managed controlled substance activities for nonclinical research. The majority of controlled substances administered to laboratory animals are utilized for euthanasia, anesthesia, and analgesia. Analytical laboratory or chemical analysis and direct research on the controlled substances themselves, either in vitro or in vivo, are additional uses for controlled substances. Additionally, many laboratory animal veterinarians have active DEA registrations and practitioner licenses. A laboratory animal veterinarian can order, store, and administer controlled substances to animals under their direct care for surgical purposes or acute medical treatment for facilities at a single location using their practitioner controlled substance license and DEA registration. The direct administration of controlled substances by veterinary technicians or animal care unit or department employees may be involved in this. All controlled substance inventory, administration, and disposal records pertaining to the medical care of laboratory animals would be kept by the veterinarian, while individual researchers or departments would keep their own state controlled substance licenses and DEA registrations for approved research.

Especially if the controlled substances will be stored at multiple separate locations within the institution, laboratory animal veterinarians are prohibited from distributing or transferring controlled substances ordered with their DEA registration to other researchers for use in research. A veterinarian may provide individual researchers with small amounts of controlled substances for anesthesia, analgesia, or euthanasia in rare instances; however, these procedures must conform to state regulations for dispensing (e.g., veterinary clinic dispensing to clients), including providing prescription instructions and keeping records. Additionally, in order to prevent and control diversion, some states mandate that all dispensed controlled substances be reported to a central database managed by the state. Consequently, laboratory animal veterinarians should refrain from dispensing or disseminating controlled substances unless approved by their state regulatory boards and the DEA.

Prevention Measures for Infections Caused by Pets and Exotic Animals

Health care professionals and veterinarians play a crucial role in educating parents and children about the dangers of owning traditional and exotic pets, as well as coming into contact with animals in public settings. Most parents and pet owners are unaware of the many ways that pets can spread zoonotic infectious diseases. Only 5% of pediatricians reported regularly educating patients or families about pet-associated salmonellosis or toxoplasmosis, despite the fact that pediatricians recognize the importance of anticipatory guidance regarding pet-related risks.[93] Pediatricians and veterinarians can remind parents, children, and pet owners of the importance of taking preventative measures. Avoiding direct contact with animals and their environments is straightforward and effective advice. This is especially crucial for sick animals, young ruminants, young poultry, reptiles, rodents, and amphibians, and animals from which the transmission of enteric pathogens is at risk. When interacting with animals in public settings, young children should always be closely supervised. Public health officials, veterinarians, animal venue operators, animal exhibitors, visitors to animal venues and exhibits, and others concerned with disease control and minimizing risks associated with animals in public settings can all benefit from the NASPHV's excellent compendium of standardized recommendations. Health care providers (HCPs) should remind pet owners to match the size and temperament of a pet to the age and behavior of an infant or child, provide direct supervision for younger children, and educate all children about proper human-animal interactions.

Parents who have children in the home frequently do not discuss their decision to acquire a nontraditional pet with HCPs or veterinarians. HCPs and veterinarians, on the other hand, are in a unique position to provide information and advice to families who already own or are considering purchasing a nontraditional pet because they are regarded as reliable sources of information regarding healthcare. Parents can be educated without significantly increasing the amount of time spent in the healthcare facility by using informational posters and brochures that can be displayed or referred to websites. Deworming, immunization, flea and tick control, diet, and physical activity can all help maintain a pet's health and reduce the likelihood of infection or injury. When parents are considering purchasing a nontraditional animal, a referral to a veterinarian can also be helpful. Veterinarians are able to provide information regarding the selection of an appropriate pet, the size of an animal when it reaches adulthood, the animal's temperament, its requirements for animal husbandry, and its suitability as a pet.

Every well-child evaluation, and especially an evaluation of a suspected infectious disease, should include a history of contact with pets in the home or animals in public settings. A history of non-traditional pets in the home or public contact with animals can prompt specific testing and additional or better treatment, and it may occasionally lead to the early identification of an unusual infection from another continent.

Welfare of Rabbits and Rodents in the Research Environment Veterinary Oversight

The laboratory animal veterinarian and the facility's animal health team play a crucial and required role in ensuring the behavioral and physical well-being of rodents and rabbits used in research. The reader is referred elsewhere for a fuller description of the expectations of an adequate veterinary care program and veterinary competency in laboratory animal medicine because it is beyond the scope of this chapter (Bayne et al., 2011; NRC, 2011). It doesn't matter how many rabbits and rodents are housed in the research facility or how big it is; all that matters is that a veterinarian who knows how to take care of rabbits and rodents' health will always be there to help with their care. Rabbits and rodents can rapidly deteriorate following the onset of illness behavior due to their small size and rapid metabolism (see Section Monitoring Animal Well-Being and Endpoint

Determination). As a result, prompt veterinary care is necessary. For certain common conditions, such as treatment for dehydration following transportation or treatment for early dermatitis, written triage procedures may be useful to reduce care delays. When receiving animals or performing routine husbandry, staff members can be instructed to recognize these states and proceed with treatment, including documentation of their actions. When it is necessary to effectively manage large rodent colonies, delegation can be beneficial. When serious conditions in animals arise that necessitate a different course of treatment, or when any questions about the animal's condition arise, the veterinarian should always be informed. According to Field et al., there are methods for keeping accurate medical records for research colonies of rabbits and rodents. 2007).

The veterinarian faces unique challenges when it comes to providing the best possible care for research rabbits and rodents. In facilities that house hundreds to thousands of animals at once, it is rare for veterinarians to be able to give each animal regular, in-depth care. Many institutions use some kind of animal incident report form to document animal injury, illness, or death in addition to delegating daily animal observations to animal caregivers and the triage of care to the animal health team. For on-study animals, these reports are typically completed by the research team or by caregivers for colony or pre-study animals. These reports can be used as educational tools to modify procedures or activities to ensure future animal well-being if they are tracked and reviewed by the veterinarian. Additionally, they are used to inform the institution's animal ethics committee of health issues that could have an effect on the welfare of research animals.

When rabbits and rodents require veterinary care, treatment carts or areas must be stocked with the appropriate equipment and supplies for their small size. Utilizing pocket-sized weigh scales, tuberculin syringes, microsurgery instruments, and 5-0 suture material, for instance, can improve dosing accuracy, treatment efficiency, and animal comfort in facilities that house and operate on mice. During examination and treatment, sick rabbits and rodents should be handled gently and quietly because they can be fragile. When dealing with medical cases involving rodents and rabbits, care must be taken to strike a balance between the demands of close monitoring the animals and the anxiety and stress that may result from frequent handling and observation. A recent review (Turner et al.,) of recommendations for routes and methods of administering medications and other substances to rabbits and rodents 2011a, b).

The laboratory animal veterinarian ought to be involved in the institutional behavioral management plans for research rodents and rabbits because behavioral well-being is also an essential component of animal health.

Finally, one important responsibility of the veterinarian in charge of monitoring the health of the research rodent and rabbit colony is establishing and maintaining an ongoing quality assurance program. As previously mentioned, the absence of disease and other debilitating conditions is not the only factor that contributes to good animal welfare; rather, it is a significant factor. Illness transmission stays normal, even in very much oversaw states, and is a specific concern when hereditarily changed rodents are divided among organizations (Carty, 2008). Understanding the dangers of agents entering a facility is necessary for the establishment of a useful monitoring program; epidemiology of parasites or microorganisms and the pathogenesis of infections; immunology, host susceptibility, and resistance; mechanisms for agent exclusion; and infection-related clinical signs.

Biomedical Animal Research and Ethics: The Vital Job of the Investigatora

P8 See your going to veterinarian as a steady wellspring of data and direction during all phases of the undertaking

Research facility creature veterinarians have skill in minimization of agony and pain and in creature lodging and care. They keep up with regulatory requirements because they are members of or advisors to IACUCs. They are familiar with various types of biomedical research, experimental methods, and their effects on research animals. During the design of the project, talking to a veterinarian can help make sure that no further changes that are required by law will be needed. By assisting in the elimination or minimization of potential harms to animals in the design or implementation of a project, veterinarians can also help ensure that the project is carried out in an ethical manner.

Occupational Health of Workers with Laboratory Animals Veterinary Staff Veterinarians who work with laboratory animals may complete internships, residencies, such as comparative medicine and pathology residencies, and further specialize in their field of practice to concentrate on the laboratory animal environment. The American College of Laboratory Animal Medicine (ACLAM) specialty board certification of veterinarians demonstrates their expertise in this field; consequently, ACLAM diplomats are frequently regarded as essential members of the occupational health team. Depending on the hiring institution and the requirements of the state, veterinary and research support technicians might or might not be licensed. Veterinary and research support staff members play a crucial role in the creation of occupational safety and health strategies for animal workers because they deal with animal diseases and the necessary animal care and handling procedures.

Principles of good prescribing practice and the responsibilities of companion animal clinicians Veterinarians are tasked with the responsibility of prescribing and dispensing drugs that are either deemed unsuitable for unrestricted availability due to particular public health considerations or cannot be used effectively or safely by laypeople. Due to their training and experience in veterinary medicine and clinical pharmacology, veterinarians are considered appropriate prescribers of these products. These obligations must be taken seriously because they are obligations and not rights.

Veterinarians are required to be aware of, comprehend, and adhere to their various legal responsibilities under applicable state, federal, national, and local laws and regulations. The authorization to practice veterinary medicine, the registration of the hospital, and the supply, use, storage, prescription, and disposal of drugs or veterinary medicines will all be included in these responsibilities. The following are some general principles of good prescribing practice and an illustration of how these principles can be applied to the appropriate use of antimicrobial agents, despite the fact that each jurisdiction has its own unique set of rules and regulations that specify the actual requirements:

Only licensed veterinarians are allowed to use or supervise the use of veterinary medicines.

Relationship between veterinarian and patient (VCPR): Veterinary medicines can only be used in conjunction with a valid VCPR if:

The client has agreed to follow the veterinarian's instructions; the veterinarian has sufficient knowledge of the animal to initiate at least a general or preliminary diagnosis of the animal's medical condition; the veterinarian is readily available for follow-up evaluation in the event of adverse reactions or treatment regimen failure; and the veterinarian has assumed responsibility for making clinical judgments regarding the patient's health and the need for medical treatment.

The US FDA's Extralabel Drug Use in Animals, 21 CFR Part 530, 9 December 1996, serves as the source for this VCPR description, which is applicable only to the United States but also serves as general guidance for other countries.

Diagnosis. Every treatment decision is based on a reliable diagnosis.

Treatment plan The development of a plan with specific treatment goals is necessary. It's helpful to think of every therapeutic intervention as a careful but thorough experiment.

Knowledge of drugs All drugs should be used in accordance with the directions on the label, unless there are compelling reasons to use them in a different way. In addition, veterinarians ought to become familiar with any additional relevant information that might make it possible to use the medication with greater safety or effectiveness.

For instance, if there is a warning about using the drug in neonatal animals, it might be found through investigation that other veterinarians have all used it safely with this kind of animal.

In a similar vein, in the event that particular organ dysfunctions are present, it may be possible to make necessary dose adjustments by looking into the literature or talking to other practitioners. Before incorporating the additional information into a therapeutic plan, it is the responsibility of the inquirer to evaluate its relevance, quality, and strength.

Communication with clients. Both to ensure that the client agrees with the decision to treat and the treatment goals, as well as to guarantee compliance with the dosage regimen, the client should be involved in the plan's development. It's important to talk about the plan's benefits and risks.

Client approval The client's informed consent should be obtained, particularly when employing an untested approach or extra-label program.

Instructions for the patient A method of administration, dose rate, frequency, and duration should be outlined in clear, understandable writing.

Product disposal and storage information ought to be provided.

The client should be encouraged to get in touch with the veterinarian who prescribed the medication if they have any questions or concerns, and any anticipated side effects should be listed in the other instructions.

Follow-up. In order to determine whether the therapeutic plan is working as expected, plans for either passive (allowing the client to call if they are concerned) or active (scheduled by the veterinarian) follow-up should be considered as appropriate.

Reassessment. The therapeutic plan's success should always be subject to objective reevaluation. There is a plethora of factors that can result in variation in clinical response to treatment, as was previously discussed in this chapter. If there is a lack of efficacy or adverse effects, these factors—such as compliance, comorbidities, and a reassessment of the diagnosis—should be systematically evaluated.

Negative events.

The manufacturer and regulatory agency should be informed of any suspected adverse events, including drug interactions.

Prescriptions.

Veterinarians must be famillar with prescription writing requirements, particularly the minimum labeling requirements (more details below). In addition, the patient's needs, the disease, the medication's expiration date, and the possibility of misuse should all be taken into consideration when determining the dosage that is prescribed.

Particular requirements Veterinarians should be aware of any breed societies, sporting organizations, or other parties' rules and regulations when prescribing medications to companion animals.

Containers.

It is preferable to distribute products in the original container with the label on it. If this is not possible, the product should ideally be dispensed in a container that is safe for children and has the appropriate information printed on it, as shown in the example below under Prescriptions.

Keep a record.

The dates of each consultation and treatment, details of drug dosage regimens, and identification of the animal treated should all be recorded in detail in a system that can be easily retrieved for the required amount of time. There may be additional record-keeping requirements for certain controlled or scheduled drugs, particularly addictive drugs.

medication storage. Medicines should be stored in accordance with applicable laws, typically in a secure location away from the general public. Each drug's storage conditions should be observed, and expired products should be removed. It is necessary to ascertain the flammability of stored goods and to take the appropriate safety precautions. It may be necessary to have bonded storage space and specific fire extinguishers in addition to separating products that are flammable and those that are not.

Getting rid of medicines. During disposal, it is essential to have knowledge of the current laws.

Antibiotics and first aid. It is prudent to be familiar with the negative effects of drug exposure on humans and animals, as well as to have the necessary first aid supplies and antidotes on hand.

The term "extra-label" or "off-label" drug use refers to the use of a drug in an animal that goes against the approved labeling. This includes using the drug in species that aren't listed on the label, using it for purposes that aren't listed on the label, and using it in dosage, frequency, or route of administration that aren't listed on the label. Utilization of an animal drug, a human-approved drug, or extemporaneous preparations can all result in extra-label use.

Extra-label use is typically restricted to situations in which an animal's health is in jeopardy, treatment failure may result in suffering or death, and no approved animal drug is available that is thought to be effective.

Extra-label drug use entails a particular set of responsibilities, including the requirement of client consent, a reasonable expectation that the chosen drug will be effective in the circumstances, and a minimum level of drug knowledge.

Prescriptions for pets should be written clearly and indelibly to prevent mistakes and ambiguity. The prescriber's jurisdiction's rules and regulations typically govern the prescription's format and content, which must be adhered to. However, the prescription typically contains the following:

date of prescription issue, prescriber's name, address, and phone number identification (name and species) of the animal(s) to be treated, as well as the name and strength of the drug(s) to be dispensed (for example, amoxicillin 100 mg): If a specific product is required, the name may be the proprietary name or the nonproprietary name if the pharmacist dispensing the prescription can choose from a selection of available products. For extemporaneous products, the dosage form and total amount to be dispensed (e.g., 25 tablets) should be included on the package label. this typically includes usage instructions (such as the route, quantity, and frequency of administration), special instructions (such as "give with food"), and warnings; Additionally, unless the signature and qualifications of the prescriber are already on the printed label of the product being dispensed, some jurisdictions require the statements "For Animal Treatment Only" and "Keep Out of the Reach of Children."

Laboratory Animal Welfare

Increasing Awareness of Laboratory Animal Welfare, It is becoming increasingly expected of veterinarians to ensure and promote animal welfare. Veterinarians are under a lot of pressure from society, both nationally and internationally, to ensure the well-being of the animals we share our lives with and use for food, work, entertainment, exhibition, education, and research. The AVMA's inclusion of animal welfare as a strategic direction for the second consecutive strategic planning period and the establishment and staffing of a Division of Animal Welfare within its headquarters that supports the AVMA's Animal

Welfare Committee (AWC) are indications of the growing recognition of this fact in the United States.

For the AVMA, the AWC develops welfare policies that address a wide range of issues, including the welfare of research animals (http://www.avma.org/issues/animal_welfare/policies. asp). The American College of Animal Welfare (ACAW) was recently established by veterinarians from many different specialties, including laboratory animal veterinarians. The AVMA recently established ACAW as a veterinary specialty organization. According to Morton (2010), "We need to convince the public that we take animal welfare seriously, and setting up a college (i.e. a specialty organization) in animal welfare is a good example of how we can that," an animal welfare board certification organization is essential for the U.S. veterinary profession. Through scientific investigation, education, and certification, the ACAW's mission is to improve animal welfare. The anesthesiology/pain management, theriogenology, poultry medicine, bovine medicine, swine medicine, equine medicine, laboratory animal medicine, companion animal medicine, zoo animal medicine, aquatic animal medicine, toxicology, internal medicine, epidemiology and public health, bioethics, and behavior experts who overlay their knowledge and expertise in animal welfare on these numerous sectors of the veterinary profession are members of the ACAW. This sends a strong message that veterinarians representing

An important step forward for animal welfare was the European Parliament's acceptance of animals as sentient beings in the Lisbon Treaty, which went into effect on December 1, 2009. The Treaty requires member states to "pay full regard to the welfare requirements of animals" (http://www.consilium.europa.eu/treaty-of-lisbon.aspx?lang=en), placing animal welfare squarely on the policy agenda for EU nations. This requirement is specific to research, technological development, and other uses of animals.

Be that as it may, for the vast majority inside those nations, the government assistance of creatures in exploration, educating, and testing was at that point an excellent thought. The Order 86/609/EEC on the security of creatures utilized for logical purposes, embraced in 1986, had set least norms for lodging and care of research facility creatures and supported the turn of events and utilization of options, bringing about laying out the ECVAM in 1991. The current review of the Directive and its replacement with the much more comprehensive EU Directive 2010/63 EU were brought about by shifting attitudes and approaches to the use of animals in science, with an increased focus on the Three Rs and the procedures for ethical review and experiment authorization. The new Directive's adoption demonstrates the European nations' dedication to animal welfare as binding legislation for all EU members. It establishes the end goal of "full replacement of procedures on live animals for scientific and educational purposes as soon as it is scientifically possible to do so" (http://eur-lex.europa.eu/LexUriServ/LexUriServ.do?uri=OJ:L:20 10:276:0033:0079:EN:PDF), which is significant and may be the first time this has been done in law.

A part-time position as Animal Welfare Coordinator was established by the NZVA in 1991 in recognition of the growing significance of animal welfare and the profession's primary focus on animal welfare (Smith, personal communication). According to Williams

(2005), the Animal Welfare Coordinator oversees the management and support of NZVA nominees to AECs as well as the development and review of animal welfare policies within the NZVA. In 2005, the NZVA's Food Safety, Animal Welfare, and Biosecurity Branch, which later changed its name to the Food Safety, Animal Welfare, and Biosecurity Branch, included animal welfare as a topic of special interest.

The NZVA launched its Animal Welfare Strategy in 2009 (http://animalwelfare.nzva.org.nz/sites/default/files/domain-44/NZVA%20Strat%20for%20web.pdf) with the goals of "respecting and recognising our members for their leadership and educational role in animal welfare and well-being" and "enabling and promoting our membership as having the knowledge, skills, and leadership in the field of animal welfare and well-being."

The current development of a national animal welfare strategy, led by MPI, has resulted from the increasing importance and awareness of animal welfare in New

Zealand as a whole. This strategy will influence the planned review of the country's animal welfare legislation. The development of the strategy is seen as an opportunity to improve and formalize existing animal welfare systems; examine the government's and other organizations' roles and responsibilities in relation to animal welfare; and cultivate a national consensus on animal welfare across all sectors, organizations, and individuals. The strategy is expected to address the changing expectations of New Zealand society regarding animal welfare.

The Australian Animal Welfare Strategy, which was launched in 2005 with the goal of improving animal welfare, highlighted Australia's importance to animal welfare. The underlying phases of the procedure were focused on six significant gatherings: animals used in education and research; companion pets; livestock farming; aquatic creatures; wildlife; and animals used for work, sport, entertainment, and display. In 2011, a second phase began, with the goal of fostering international partnerships for animal welfare. The Animal Welfare Committee of the Australian Veterinary Association (AVA) is in charge of the Association's numerous animal welfare policies.

Additionally, the AVA has established an Animal Welfare Trust to support and promote animal welfare research and education for all species of animals, including pets, farm and laboratory animals, wildlife, and zoo animals.

Since 2000, ANZCVS has had an Animal Welfare Chapter in recognition of the increasingly specialized role that veterinarians play in the field of animal welfare science. Its members include veterinarians who work in animal research settings as well as practitioners and government employees.

The series of World Congresses for Alternatives and Animal Use in the Life Sciences has played a significant role in raising awareness of animal welfare within the research and testing communities. Since the first congress, which was held in Baltimore in 1993 and was organized by the Johns Hopkins CAAT, these congresses have been held every two to three years. 2011 saw the eighth meeting take place in Montreal. The meetings have attracted a large number of stakeholders, scientists, veterinarians, and animal welfare organizations interested in scientific approaches to the development and use of methods that replace, reduce, and/or refine (the Three Rs) animal-based laboratory methods. The specific focus is on the Three Rs in relation to the use of animals in research, teaching, and testing. The diverse backgrounds of the participants are demonstrated by the long list of sponsors, which has included pharmaceutical, chemical, and cosmetic companies; groups that protect animals; associations for science and laboratory animals; associations for animals; and academic institutions.

Animals with Influenza A

Viruses Many different kinds of animals, such as ducks, chickens, pigs, horses, seals, and cats, carry influenza A virus.

Influenza B viruses only affect humans and are highly contagious.

Based on the presence of two proteins on the surface of the virus, influenza A viruses are divided into subtypes: the neuraminidase (N) and the hemagglutinin. (H) There are 11 distinct neuraminidase subtypes and 18 distinct hemagglutinin subtypes. Except for subtypes H17N10 and H18N11, which have only been found in bats, all of the known subtypes of influenza A viruses have been found in birds.

Although it is uncommon for humans to contract influenza directly from animals, certain avian influenza A viruses have been linked to isolated human infections and outbreaks.

What exactly is the bat flu?

The influenza A viruses in bats are referred to as "bat flu." Bat influenza was first found in "minimal yellow-bore bats" in Guatemala during a review led in 2009 and 2010 by specialists from CDC and the Universidad del Valle (College of the Valley) in Guatemala (1). Since then, bat flu viruses have been found in other bat species in Central and South America (2). According to laboratory research conducted at the CDC and elsewhere, these viruses would need to undergo significant modifications before they could easily infect humans and spread. The bat species that are currently known to carry bat flu are prevalent in Central and South America, not the continental United States.

Is human health at risk from bat flu?

According to preliminary CDC laboratory research, bat flu viruses cannot grow in a test tube on human cells. This suggests that the bat flu virus might not grow or reproduce in humans and would need to change a lot for them to be able to easily infect and spread among humans. However, due to the fact that testing of the bat flu virus's genome reveals that its internal genes are compatible with those of human flu viruses, the researchers at the CDC are unable to rule out the possibility that these viruses will one day be able to infect humans. The question titled "How could bat flu viruses become capable of infecting and spreading among humans?" provides additional information.

How did the bat flu virus become capable of infecting humans and spreading?

It is possible that bat flu viruses and human flu viruses could share genetic information through a process known as "reassortment" because their internal genes are compatible with one another. When two or more flu viruses infect a single host cell, reassortment occurs, allowing the viruses to swap their genetic information. Reassortment can occasionally result in the emergence of new human-infectible influenza viruses.

However, it is still unknown what conditions are necessary for human and bat flu viruses to reassort. An alternate creature (like pigs, ponies, canines or seals) would have to act as a "span," implying that such a creature would should be equipped for being tainted with both this new bat seasonal infection and human seasonal infections for reassortment to happen. At least one study has looked into the possibility of bat flu reassortment with other flu viruses since the virus was first discovered (3). The findings of these studies continue to suggest that bat flu viruses are very unlikely to recombine with other flu viruses to produce new viruses that could be more dangerous or infectious. The bat flu viruses appear to not be a threat to human health in their current form.

What is the significance of the bat flu discovery for public health?

Because bats are a novel animal species that may serve as a source of flu viruses, the discovery of bat flu is significant for public health. It is already known that influenza viruses infect domestic and wild birds, pigs, horses, and dogs, as well as occasionally infect seals, whales, ferrets, and cats. Because the previous pandemics of the 20th century as well as the 2009 H1N1 pandemic were caused by flu viruses in animals that gained the ability to infect and spread easily to humans, the CDC and disease experts around the world monitor flu viruses that circulate in animals.

What can we learn about flu viruses from the discovery of bat flu?

The evolution of influenza A, B, and C viruses has been illuminated by the discovery of bat flu. It is possible that many of the internal genes of bat influenza viruses come from families of flu viruses that used to be more common in earlier centuries but are now extinct or have yet to be found. Phylogenic analysis, a method used to compare the various bat flu viruses found in Central and South America, has revealed that these viruses have a lot of genetic variation. Some flu researchers came to the conclusion that the bat flu viruses found in Central and South American bat populations may have as much genetic diversity in some gene segments as the flu viruses of all other mammal and bird species taken together. This indicates that these viruses have been evolving in bats for extremely long periods of time, possibly for centuries.

What distinguishes the bat flu virus from other flu viruses?

The bat flu viruses found in Central and South America differ significantly from other human and animal flu viruses. Hemagglutinin (HA) surface proteins are present in all flu A viruses. Prior to the discovery of these viruses, there were only 16 distinct classes (or "subtypes") of HA proteins that were known to exist in nature. The CDC has designated the new bat flu viruses discovered in Central and South America as new subtypes with the designations "H17" and "H18" because they are sufficiently distinct from the previously identified subtypes (1, 2). Neuraminidase (NA), the other surface protein-coding gene of bat flu viruses, differs significantly from that of known flu viruses. This gene could have come from ancient bat flu viruses that are either no longer in existence or have yet to be discovered. The NA subtypes that are found in bats have been given new names by scientists at the CDC: N10" and "N11."

Does the bat flu virus's surface protein structure differ from that of humans?

According to flu researchers, the bat flu virus's HA and NA surface proteins perform a different function than those of human, other mammal, and bird flu viruses. HA surface proteins, for instance, make it possible for the flu virus to attach to and enter a human respiratory tract cell, which is how infection occurs in humans. In a similar manner, the NA surface proteins that are found on flu viruses that infect humans, birds, and other mammals also play a role in infection because they enable a flu virus to escape an infected cell and infect a different cell that is not infected. An examination of the crystal structures of the bat flu viruses in Central and South America reveals, however, that the HA and NA proteins do not carry out these tasks in the same manner. The researchers came to the conclusion that the bats must have a distinct mechanism of action for these surface proteins. As a result, it is currently unknown how these bat flu viruses enter or exit cells to infect bats.

H7N2 Questions and Answers Although cats can be wonderful companions; their owners should be aware that they may be carriers of germs that can infect humans. Keep in mind that even healthy-looking cats can transmit infectious diseases to humans and other animals. After handling cats, cleaning a litter box, or coming into contact with cat saliva or feces, you should always wash your hands with soap and running water. It is possible to lessen the likelihood of disease transmission between people and their pets by thoroughly washing your hands. At Healthy Pets,

Healthy People, you can find additional guidance on how to maintain one's health while enjoying one's cat. Cats.

Who is H7N2?

The influenza virus H7N2 typically infects birds. Despite the fact that avian influenza viruses, more commonly referred to as "bird flu" or "avian flu," rarely infect humans, human infection has occurred in the past. Humans typically contract the bird flu virus after coming into direct contact with infected birds.

Is my cat infected with H7N2?

Only cats associated with New York City's animal shelters—specifically, the Animal Care Centers of New York City's (ACC) shelters—have been found to be infected with H7N2. In the United States, no other H7N2 outbreaks or infections of cats with H7N2 have been reported. Therefore, unless your cat recently entered an ACC animal shelter in New York City, there is very little chance that he or she has H7N2.

How do cats catch the influenza virus?

While human seasonal influenza viruses have been reported to occasionally infect cats, avian influenza infections, such as those caused by infected poultry, are known but uncommon. However, feline influenza can spread through direct contact (licking, nuzzling) in the same manner as human influenza. through the air (including nasal discharge and coughing or sneezing droplets); and by touching contaminated surfaces (such as cages, water bowls, or food bowls). Additionally, the germs in cat saliva may be transferred to the cat's coat during grooming, can contaminate the pet's environment and spread to people through contact (e.g., petting, kissing).

How can a cat transmit the flu virus to a person?

In most cases, a person can get the flu if enough of the virus gets into their eyes, nose, or mouth or is inhaled (from virus-laden droplets or dust). By touching a sick cat's eyes, nose, or mouth with virus-laden secretions, people could potentially contract the flu. Likewise, debilitated felines might hack or sniffle, which can remove drops containing the infection very high that an individual can take in or that can enter an individual's eyes, nose or mouth.

How do cats experience influenza symptoms?

Although it is uncommon, influenza infections in cats typically cause mild illness. Although not all sick cats exhibit symptoms, cats infected with the influenza virus may exhibit the following signs and symptoms of respiratory illness:

Sneezing, coughing, fever, discharge from the nose or eyes, lack of energy, and a lack of appetite are symptoms of influenza in cats. Other complications, such as pneumonia or secondary bacterial infections, may also occur. During the current outbreak in NYC animal shelters, cats infected with the H7N2 influenza virus have also displayed persistent cough, lip smacking, runny nose, and fever.

How come the CDC is worried about H7N2?

Changes in flu viruses that are found in both human and animal populations are monitored by the CDC as part of its mission to safeguard the public from emerging health threats. It is always troubling to discover the bird flu virus in an unexpected animal, like a cat, because this indicates that the virus has changed in a way that may pose a new health risk. Animal viruses that can infect humans are especially worrying because most people don't already have an immune system that can stop them. Also, if a new animal virus can infect humans and spread quickly from one person to another, it could lead to a pandemic, which is an international outbreak of disease. To prevent the novel virus from spreading to more people, these incidents need to be thoroughly investigated and the necessary steps taken.

Is there a vaccine for H7N2 in humans? Will the flu shot I get this season protect me from H7N2?

No, there is not yet a human vaccine that can protect against this virus, and neither does the flu vaccine for this season. In the event of an emergency, the U.S. pandemic preparedness stockpile contains a candidate vaccine virus (CVV) that could be provided to manufacturers of flu vaccine for mass production of a H7N2 vaccine. The CDC will test this H7N2 CVV to see if it provides protection from the 2016 H7N2 virus.

Is there a way to treat someone who has the H7N2 virus?

Yes, flu antiviral medications are used to treat seasonal flu in children and adults, and based on what we know so far about the H7N2 virus, the recommended and approved medications should work.

Early treatment has been shown to be more effective in other flu viruses, and it is especially important for people who are more likely to experience complications from the flu.

Which groups are particularly susceptible to serious flu-related complications?

The CDC is of the opinion that people who are at risk for complications from the seasonal flu would also be at risk for severe illness from H7N2. Among these are the following: people over 65, pregnant women, people with certain long-term health conditions (such as asthma, diabetes, heart disease, weakened immune systems, and neurological or neurodevelopmental conditions), children younger than 5 years old, especially those under 2 years old,

At People at High Risk of Developing Flu-Related Complications, you can find a comprehensive list of people who are at risk of developing flu-related complications.

Depending on their severity, flu complications may necessitate hospitalization or even death. Therefore, if your pet has flu symptoms, you should not allow it to kiss or lick your face. If your pet has a flu-like illness, you should avoid cuddling with it.

Can my cat transmit H7N2?

You can't get H7N2 from your cat if it doesn't have it. If your cat is infected with H7N2, there is a low chance that you will get H7N2 from coming into contact with your cat, but the risk is likely to go up the longer and more intensely you are exposed.

Can I contract H7N2 even if I avoid contact with cats?

The CDC is of the opinion that there is a very low risk of H7N2 infection for individuals who have not come into contact with infected cats based on what is currently known.

What is the dog flu, or canine influenza?

Canine influenza, also known as "dog flu," is a respiratory illness that can spread to dogs and is brought on by certain Type A influenza viruses that are known to infect dogs. These are known as "viruses of the canine influenza." There have never been any human cases of canine influenza reported. There are two distinct flu A canine seasonal infection: The H3N8 virus and the H3N2 virus are the two types. Seasonal influenza A(H3N2) viruses, which infect humans annually, are distinct from canine influenza A(H3N2) viruses.

Can humans be infected by canine influenza viruses?

It is generally believed that canine influenza viruses pose little risk to humans. There is currently no evidence that the canine influenza virus has spread from dogs to humans, and neither the United States nor any other country has reported a single case of human infection with the canine influenza virus.

But influenza viruses change all the time, and a canine influenza virus could change to be able to infect humans and easily spread from one person to another. When human infections with novel (new, non-human) influenza A viruses occur, which the human population has limited immunity to, the potential for a pandemic is cause for concern. As a result, human infections caused by novel influenza A viruses of animal origin (such as avian or swine influenza A viruses) have been identified by the global surveillance system of the World Health Organization; however, human infections caused by canine influenza A viruses have not yet been identified.

How long have canine influenza viruses existed and where did they originate?

The H3N8 canine influenza virus was first found in horses, then spread to dogs, and now it can spread between dogs. Since more than 40 years ago, it has been known that horses are infected with the H3N8 equine influenza (horse flu) virus. In 2004, the United States received reports of cases of an unidentified respiratory illness in dogs—at first, greyhounds. Equine influenza A(H3N8) viruses were found to be the cause of this respiratory illness, according to an investigation. Researchers believe that this virus evolved from horses to dogs and has adapted to infect dogs and spread to other dogs, particularly those kept in kennels and shelters. This is now regarded as a canine-specific H3N8 virus. Experts classified this virus as a "newly emerging pathogen in the dog population" in the United States in September 2005. It has now been found in dogs in a significant portion of the United States.

The H3N2 canine influenza virus was first found in birds, then spread to dogs, and now it can spread between dogs. Additionally, it has been reported that infected dogs can transmit H3N2 canine influenza viruses to cats. In 2007, the canine influenza A H3N2 virus was first found in dogs in South Korea. Since then, dogs have also been found in China, Thailand, and Canada. In April 2015, the H3N2 canine influenza virus was first observed in the United States. Since then, it has been observed in more than 30 states. The H3N2 canine viruses that have been discovered in the United States so far are nearly identical in genetic makeup to those that have only been discovered in Asia.

How does the problem of canine influenza affect dogs brought into the United States from other nations?

In the United States, these two canine influenza viruses—H3N8 and H3N2—are now considered endemic. In addition, there is currently no evidence that canine influenza can spread to humans or cause a pandemic. CDC regulations require that dogs be healthy to enter the United States; consequently, dogs may be denied entry or further evaluated if they appear to be sick with a communicable disease such as canine influenza. If there was evidence that canine influenza viruses were able to infect people with the potential for sustained human-to-human spread, CDC would exercise its existing authority to limit the introduction and/or spread of that pandemic strain either into or within the United States. For dogs that appear to be sick, the CDC may request a veterinary examination at the owner's expense or a necropsy (animal autopsy) upon arrival in the United States.

How is the CDC dealing with canine influenza?

Only viruses with the potential to cause a pandemic in humans are subject to the regulations that are currently in place at the CDC for influenza viruses. However, in the unlikely event that canine influenza becomes a threat to humans or other animals, the CDC is taking a number of precautions. First, all human infections with novel influenza A viruses are thoroughly investigated, and the CDC maintains year-round surveillance for seasonal and novel influenza A viruses. The CDC accepts reports of human infection with an animal-derived novel influenza A virus; Canine influenza viruses have not yet been linked to any human infections. Second, in the event of an outbreak of novel influenza A viruses, the CDC and USDA APHIS VS already have collaborative protocols in place. In the event of an outbreak of canine influenza with potential human infections, these same procedures would be followed. Thirdly, utilizing the Influenza Risk Assessment Tool, the CDC assessed the pandemic potential of canine H3N2 viruses and determined that it was low risk.

What symptoms does canine influenza present in dogs?

Cough, runny nose, fever, lethargy, eye discharge, and decreased appetite are symptoms of this illness in dogs; however, not all dogs will exhibit these symptoms. The severity of canine flu symptoms in dogs can range from no symptoms to severe illness that can lead to pneumonia and even death.

Within two to three weeks, most dogs recover. Notwithstanding, a few canines might foster optional bacterial contaminations which might prompt more serious disease and pneumonia. Contact your veterinarian if you have any questions about your pet's health or if they are showing symptoms of canine influenza.

The term "avian influenza" refers to a disease in birds brought on by infection with Type A avian influenza viruses. Over a hundred distinct species of wild birds from around the world have been found to be infected with avian influenza A viruses. These viruses can infect domestic poultry and other bird and animal species and are naturally found in wild aquatic birds all over the world. Waterfowl (ducks, geese, swans, gulls, and terns) and shorebirds (storks, plovers, and sandpipers) are examples of wild aquatic birds. Avian influenza A viruses are thought to be reservoirs (hosts) in wild aquatic birds, especially dabbling ducks. The intestines and respiratory tracts of wild aquatic birds can be infected with avian influenza A viruses, but some species, like ducks, may not become ill. However, avian influenza A viruses are highly contagious among birds, and certain domesticated bird species, such as chickens, ducks, and turkeys, can be sickened or even eradicated by these viruses.

Avian influenza A viruses can be shed by infected birds through their saliva, nasal secretions, and feces. When susceptible birds come into contact with the virus as it is shed by infected birds, they become infected. Additionally, they may contract the disease by coming into contact with surfaces that have been infected with the virus from infected birds.

What is equine influenza, also known as the horse flu?

The nose, throat, and occasionally the lungs are affected by horse flu, also known as equine influenza. Influenza viruses are the culprits, and they typically infect horses as well as closely related animals like donkeys and zebras. These animals exhibit flu-like signs and symptoms, similar to those experienced by people with seasonal influenza.

Initially, the "horse flu" virus spread from birds to horses. Historically, horse flu viruses, also known as "equine influenza viruses" (abbreviated EIV), were Type A influenza viruses with two subtypes: H3N8 and H7N7

The EIV H7N7 subtype was first described in the 1950s, and its last description was made in the 1970s. It is currently thought to be extinct.

In the 1960s, the EIV H3N8 subtype was first identified in horses in the United States, and it continues to spread worldwide to horses today.

Dogs, horses, and birds all carry a subtype of the H3N8 virus, but the viruses are distinct from one another.

Can the horse flu affect humans?

Horse flu viruses have been shown to be able to infect people in experimental settings, and a few people who have come into contact with infected horses have developed antibodies to the virus—a sign of infection—but no people who have been exposed to the virus have become ill, according to the World Organization for Animal Health. Horse flu viruses generally do not pose a significant threat to humans. Despite the fact that horse flu viruses are currently not well adapted to humans, it is possible that one of these viruses will one day change in such a way that it will be able to easily infect and spread among humans. Because of this, the CDC and its partners in animal health closely monitor the evolution of the flu viruses that are in circulation. This kind of surveillance is especially important for keeping track of changes to the flu viruses in animals that could spread to humans.

The avian flu A(H3N8) continues to infect birds, but these viruses are distinct from those that infect horses. Human infections with avian (bird) flu A(H3N8) viruses have been reported worldwide in the past and recently, although they are uncommon. In the late 1990s, EIV H3N8 evolved into a canine influenza virus as it spread to dogs in the United States. It was last reported in 2016, indicating that dogs no longer carry this virus.

How does horse flu spread from one horse to another?

It is thought that droplets produced when a horse coughs or sneezes spread the horse flu virus, which is highly contagious among horses. The virus can then enter the eyes, nose, or mouth, or other horses nearby can breathe it in. Currently, horse flu viruses are not well-suited for human infection.

EIV can be shed by horses even before they show symptoms of illness. Horse flu viruses can also spread through items with the virus on them, like brushes, equipment, and clothing. The virus could spread if a susceptible horse inhales, absorbs, or ingests virus from an object. Additionally, surfaces where infected animals are housed or transported can harbor EIV.

It is essential to limit access to individuals who have not been exposed during an outbreak and to practice good infection control and hygiene measures in herds, such as washing one's hands and clothing. Within one to three days, horses typically exhibit signs of the horse flu infection. It has the potential to rapidly spread and cause significant outbreaks among horses once it is introduced into an area with a population of animals that are susceptible. Spread among animals is made more likely by factors like crowding and transportation.

Can horses and other mammals be infected with the equine influenza virus?

The virus that causes horse flu first infects horses from birds. Horses were infected by avian influenza A(H3N8) viruses that circulated in birds. These viruses eventually adapted to horses and began regularly spreading as equine influenza A(H3N8) viruses in horses. 1963 marked the first time these viruses were isolated from horses. Exposure to infected animal saliva and mucus can result in infection.

EIV H3N8 became infected with canine influenza A (H3N8) virus at the end of the 1990s, when it adapted to dogs and began spreading frequently through them. The H3N8 viruses in dogs, horses, and birds all developed distinct characteristics as they became adapted to their respective hosts. The canine influenza H3N8 virus is now extinct, whereas other H3N8 viruses continue to spread in horses and birds.

How did horses get horse flu into dogs?

After spreading to dogs and adapting to them, EIV H3N8 evolved into canine influenza virus H3N8, which is now extinct in dogs. In 2004, the United States received reports of cases of an unknown illness in dogs—at first, greyhounds—affecting the nose, throat, and occasionally the lungs. Equine influenza A(H3N8) viruses were found to be the cause of this illness, according to an investigation. Researchers hypothesize that this virus spread from horses to dogs and adapted to infect and spread among dogs, particularly those kept in kennels and shelters. Human CIV H3N8 infections were not reported. In dogs, CIV H3N8 is now extinct.

What signs do horses with horse flu exhibit?

EIV-infected horses may have a dry cough and a fever (body temperature between 39 and 41 degrees Celsius). Horses with severe illness may wheeze when breathing. There may also be other symptoms like a lack of appetite, tiredness, and a runny nose. Horses that have received the EIV vaccine, which is available in the United States, may not exhibit any of these symptoms.

Is there a horse flu vaccine available?

Since the 1970s, horse flu vaccines have been available for purchase. They include the horse flu viruses that spread the most frequently and are associated with various vaccines and vaccine viruses. These vaccines are frequently utilized for the vaccination of domestic horses. An expert panel from the World Organization for Animal Health frequently proposes which viruses should be included in vaccines.

What is swine flu? What are the most important facts about it?

Swine influenza, or swine flu, is a respiratory illness that affects pigs and is brought on by the type A influenza virus, which frequently causes pigs to get the flu. Human infections of the swine flu virus are uncommon, but they have occurred. See Variant Influenza Viruses in Humans for additional information regarding human swine influenza infections.) Pig seasonal infections can cause elevated degrees of sickness in pig crowds, yet objective few passings in pigs. Although swine influenza viruses can spread throughout the year, most outbreaks occur in the late fall and winter, just like in humans.

How many viruses are there in the swine flu?

Swine flu viruses are constantly evolving, just like influenza viruses in humans and other animals. Swine influenza viruses as well as avian influenza and human influenza viruses can infect pigs. New viruses that are a mix of swine, human, and/or avian influenza viruses can emerge when influenza viruses from different species infect pigs. This process is known as reassortment, and it involves swapping genes. Various strains of the swine flu virus have emerged over time. There are currently three primary subtypes of the influenza A virus that have been isolated from pigs in the United States: H3N2, H1N1, and others

How does pig swine flu spread?

It is believed that pigs spread swine flu viruses primarily through close contact and possibly through the transfer of contaminated objects between infected and uninfected pigs. Swine herds that are infected, including those that have been vaccinated against swine flu, may only exhibit mild or no symptoms of the disease.

What symptoms do pigs have of the swine flu?

Fever, depression, coughing (barking), discharge from the nose or eyes, sneezing, difficulty breathing, eye redness or inflammation, and not eating are all symptoms of swine flu in pigs. However, some influenza-infected pigs may not exhibit any symptoms at all.

How prevalent is pig swine flu?

The swine flu viruses H1N1 and H3N2 are prevalent in American pig populations, and the industry routinely deals with them. Episodes among pigs ordinarily happen in colder climate months (pre-winter and winter), yet can happen all year. H3N2 influenza viruses did not begin to infect pigs in the United States until around 1998, whereas H1N1 swine viruses have been known to infect pig populations since at least 1930. Humans were the first to introduce the H3N2 viruses to the pig population.

However, the H3N2 viruses that were circulating in pigs have changed since then. The current H3N2 viruses that are present in pigs are vastly distinct from the seasonal H3N2 viruses that are present in humans.

Is there a swine flu vaccine available?

There are specific swine influenza vaccines available, just like there are influenza vaccines for humans.

Made in United States
Troutdale, OR
05/17/2024